The purpose of thi
book is to inspire an
   brighter, shinier pe
Take from it what you need. Go page
by page or flick to a page and see if it
provides some wisdom or insight. Its all
words, quotes, books, authors and stuff
that has made me laugh, think deeper
or differently over the years. The space
is for your to write, doodle or put other
quotes in that inspire you. I hope it
helps you to smile more on stormy days
and helps you to find whatever is
already inside of you.

Shine bright you beautiful goddess

Love and blessings

Nicola x

Never stop believing that amazing things can happen to you - especially in the most challenging times.

Important life lesson - Part 1
You cannot make people like you,
love you, accept you or make
them see things from the same
perspective as you. You cannot
control them either.

Part 2 - None of part 1 matters. How you feel about you and how you like, love and accept yourself is THE most important thing.

Put on your favourtie song - the one that makes you feel like dancing - DANCE!

Send a message to a friend that you haven't spoken to in a while.

If you see something in someone today - tell them about it. It may be their hair, or their lovely yellow coat, or just that they look happy. Acknowledge it.
By noticing something in them - YOU may just make their day.

Read "UNTAMED" by Glennon Doyle -
it will be a life changing read.

Go outside tonight and look up at the stars - you are made of the same stuff - STARDUST!

Post something that inspires you on your social media. It may inspire someone else.

Notice when your feeling good today! pay attention to what your doing and who you are with - spend more time there.

Re-watch your favourite disney movie - or one you have never watched. A guaranteed lift for your soul.

You are beautiful, unique and perfectly you. Remember this the next time your 'thoughts' are telling you otherwise.

Google 'inspiring women' and read some of their wise words. It may be just what you need to hear today.

If today feels like its going to be a tough day, remember that tough times ALWAYS pass.

Your dreams are YOURS - no one in the entire universe will ever have a dream like yours. Step into them, who knows where they will take you!

EVERYTHING you experience comes from inside of you. YOU create your life! Make it a happy, bright vibrant one.

YOUR imagination is your only limit on creating a life that you LOVE.

You are amazing!
Find an affirmation that you love
for yourself

Life is like a big squiggly graph. Its full of highs and lows and lots of in-betweens. Find your calm for the in-betweens.

Listen to an inspiring podcast.
I love Fearne Cotton, Oprah.

Celebrate your wins today!
No matter how small.

Everyday is a NEW day.
Remember that if
yesterday was particularly
terrible.

Its never about what you have or how you look or what you achieve. The most important things about you are the way you love, your courage and your energy. That's what other people remember.

The secret to being 'Shiny' is noticing the everyday magic in your life. The extra squishy hug you get from a child, The way your coffee tastes when you get to drink it in peace and an unexpected check-in from a friend. Noticing these 'magic' moments make the world more 'magical'.

Be bold, be kind, give generously, speak truly and from the heart. Be brave, BE YOU.

Treat yourself to your favourite indulgence today. A fancy coffee and some cake. A new lippy. YOU deserve it.

All those thoughts, worries and anxieties that you have are covering up how you 'SHINE in the world. Find a way to put them all down and notice how brighter you feel.

If its not going to matter this time next year, try not to worry about it so much today.

Create a 'Shine' doodle.

We are what we think. All that we are arises with our thoughts. With our thoughts, WE make the world.
BUDDHA

Try shifting your perspective when thoughts of your past come up. Focus on how far you have come, what you have achieved and how it has shaped you into becoming YOU.

Some see a wish, some see a weed. It's all about your own perspective.

Someday. Oneday. Maybe.
They are all just thoughts. However,
if you take steps towards them, they
may just become your reality.

A heart full of love and a head full of good thoughts, will never go wrong.

Happiness is only ever one thought away, but you must find for yourself that ONE thought.
Syd Banks

Surround yourself with people who see your light, your worth and your potential. Especially if you cannot see these things for yourself.

Do something that makes your heart happy today. Sing, Dance, Bake or clean the kitchen. Whatever works for you.

Love people exactly as they are. Then watch how they SHINE and GROW.

Take some time out today to notice
all the amazing things that you
have already brought into your life

Find your CALM, the thing that sees you through all of life's challenges. A lovely bath, a book or coffee with a great friend.

YOU BE YOU

We are all just learning how to navigate ourselves through this life. Our mistakes, wrong turns and challenges will be our greatest lessons.

Smile for no reason today!

Eat something you love. Cake, Avocados, Celery - just do it without any judgement.

Set your WEIRDNESS free - let it out, you will find all your fellow weirdos that way!!

Remember that you cannot and do not have to do it all alone. Rest. Recharge. Ask for help before you fall.

We are all different. We all have our own unique view of life - that's what makes it so interesting!!

Fill your head with good thoughts, compliment yourself - embrace your uniqueness. You spend so much time there - Enjoy it!

Do something thats on your To-do List! You will have an instant sense of achievement!

If your feeling overwhelmed today, take small actions until you feel calmer.

Sometimes life is all about joy
and hopes and dreams.
Sometimes its just about focusing
on the next step. All of this is OK.
Just as long as its the right next
step for you.

Be brave enough to ask for
help when you need it.

If your going through a storm just now, remember. One day, you will look back and wonder where you found the strength to make it through and be amazed at how it didn't break you. You wont have came out of that storm the same person. In your storms YOU can find your strength.

Maybe you don't have all your ducks in a row just yet. Maybe you have sloths at a spa or squirrels at a rave. Just enjoy where you are NOW.

"My darling girl, when are you going to realise that being normal is not necessarily a virtue. It rather denotes a lack of courage!"
Aunt Francis
Practical Magic (my fave movie)

I wish I could show you when
you are lonely or in darkness,
the astonishing light of your
own being.
Hafiz

What do you share about yourself
that truly comes from the heart?

Who would you be if you embraced all your uniqueness? What would your life look and feel like? What experience would you be having?

There is no force more powerfull
than a woman, determined to rise!
W.E.B Dubois

Who do you admire? Who inspires you? Think about what qualities they have that makes them SHINE!

"Am gan roon the bend - thank
christ a ken my wiy hame"
Keri Burnett
your heart will always lead you
home - no matter how crazy life
feels in the moment

The stories we cling to depend on what perspective we see them from.

Just for today - experience the joy of living in the present moment!

Let the waters settle and you will
see the moon and the stars mirrored
in your own being.
RUMI

You are an amazingly beautiful,
magical human being!

You look amazing!
Have you lost weight?
I love your outfit!
(Take a compliment for yourself)

What lens are you viewing life through today?
Happy - Sad - Joyful - Anxious
Which one gives you the best day?

If you dont believe in magic, how will you ever experience it?

Find your own way of
bringing peace to your heart.
Life will become so much
MORE!

Spend some time in your
favourite place today!

Make a Space in your home for
HYGGE - Just for you!
(Danish idea - amazingly nurturing
for you)

Sometimes, life will knock you down.
Get back up as soon as you can

WISDOM

Stop. Breathe. Then respond.
Best not to jump in
Jackie Gillespie
(The Listening Space)

Give meditation a try. There are so many ways. Use an app, try a guided one. Use a mantra. Do a shaking meditation. There is definitely one for you.

Its OK to change.
your mind, Your heart, Your
direction
If it doesn't bring you joy -
change it!

The story of your life is yours to write.
Dream Big.
Laugh hard.
Find the joy in everyday,
it will be an epic tale

Printed in Great Britain
by Amazon

54213935R00045